BOOK 2

Elevate Your Potential:

A Guide to Personal Growth and Success

ISBN: 9798334644885

by- *Arya Gupta*

Year of publishing- 2024

Cover design by *Arya Gupta*

ISBN: 9798334644885

Published by Self-Published

For permissions or inquiries, contact:
iaryaguptaa@example.com

First Edition, July 2024

Printed in the INDIA

Preface

Welcome to "Elevate Your Potential: A Guide to Personal Growth and Success." This book is the culmination of my journey, insights, and experiences in the realm of personal development. My hope is that it serves as a practical guide and a source of inspiration for anyone looking to unlock their potential and achieve their dreams.

The idea for this book was born out of a personal quest for growth and improvement. Like many of you, I have faced challenges, setbacks, and moments of self-doubt. Through these experiences, I discovered the importance of understanding and harnessing one's potential. I realized that the key to personal and professional success lies within each of us, waiting to be unlocked.

In writing this book, I aimed to create a comprehensive and accessible resource that anyone can use to embark on their journey of self-discovery and growth. Each chapter is designed to provide you with actionable strategies, real-life examples, and practical exercises that you can implement immediately. Whether you're looking to improve your habits, set and achieve meaningful goals, or develop a growth mindset, this book offers tools and insights to help you on your way.

One of the most rewarding aspects of personal development is the realization that the journey is ongoing. There is always room for growth, learning, and improvement. As you read through these pages, I encourage you to embrace this mindset. Approach each chapter with an open heart and a willingness to apply what you learn. Remember, the path to success is not a straight line but a series of steps, each bringing you closer to your true potential.

I would like to extend my gratitude to everyone who has supported me on this journey. Your encouragement and belief in my vision have been instrumental in bringing this book to life. To my readers, thank you for choosing this book as a companion on your journey. I am honored to be a part of your quest for growth and success.

Finally, I invite you to connect with me and share your experiences. Your stories, feedback, and insights are invaluable, not only to me but to the entire community of readers who are on similar paths. Together, we can inspire and support each other in reaching new heights.

Thank you for allowing me to be a part of your journey. I hope you find "Elevate Your Potential: A Guide to Personal Growth and Success" to be a valuable and transformative resource.

Warm regards,

Arya Gupta

`Introduction: Elevate Your Potential

Setting the Stage

Welcome to "Elevate Your Potential: A Guide to Personal Growth and Success." This book is your trusted companion on a transformative journey toward unlocking your true potential and achieving the success you desire. Whether you're seeking to improve your personal life, enhance your professional career, or cultivate a sense of overall well-being, the principles and strategies within these pages are designed to guide you every step of the way.

In today's fast-paced world, it's easy to feel overwhelmed and stuck. Many of us go through life without realizing the vast reservoir of potential we carry within. We get caught up in daily routines, external expectations, and self-imposed limitations, often losing sight of our true capabilities and aspirations. This book aims to help you break free from those limitations, recognize the power you possess, and provide you with the tools needed to achieve your dreams.

Purpose of the Book

The purpose of this book is simple yet profound: to help you elevate your life. We live in a world full of opportunities, but often, our potential remains untapped due to self-doubt, lack of direction, or external obstacles. This book aims to break those barriers and empower you with the knowledge and tools to pursue your goals confidently and effectively.

You'll find practical advice, real-life examples, and actionable strategies that you can apply immediately to start making positive changes in your life. This isn't just a book to read—it's a guide to implement. By engaging with the content and practicing the exercises provided, you'll be able to see tangible progress and growth in various aspects of your life.

What to Expect

Each chapter of this book delves into a critical aspect of personal growth. From understanding your potential and cultivating the right mindset to setting achievable goals and overcoming obstacles, every section is packed with actionable advice, real-life examples, and practical exercises. By the end of this book, you'll have a comprehensive roadmap to elevate your potential and sustain your success.

Here's a brief overview of what we'll cover:

1. **Understanding Potential**: Learn what potential truly means, how to recognize it within yourself, and why it's important to unlock it.
2. **Mindset and Motivation**: Discover the power of a growth mindset and find techniques to stay motivated and overcome self-doubt.

3. **Goal Setting and Planning**: Master the art of setting SMART goals and creating actionable plans to achieve them.
4. **Building Positive Habits**: Understand the science of habits and learn how to build and maintain positive routines.
5. **Overcoming Obstacles**: Equip yourself with strategies to handle setbacks and learn from failures.
6. **Leveraging Strengths and Skills**: Identify your unique strengths and learn how to apply them effectively in your personal and professional life.
7. **Creating a Supportive Environment**: Build a network of positive influences and manage negative environments.
8. **Sustaining Growth and Success**: Develop long-term strategies for continuous improvement and celebrate your achievements.

The Journey Begins

Embracing Change

Change is an inevitable part of life. While it can be daunting, it's also a powerful catalyst for growth. Embracing change means being open to new experiences, learning opportunities, and the evolution of your own potential. Throughout this book, you'll be encouraged to step out of your comfort zone, challenge your assumptions, and embrace the changes necessary for your personal development.

Change is not always easy. It requires courage, perseverance, and a willingness to face uncertainty. But it's through these challenges that we grow the most. As you embark on this journey, remember that every step forward, no matter how small, brings you closer to unlocking your full potential.

The Power of Mindset

At the core of personal growth is your mindset. How you perceive yourself and the world around you significantly impacts your ability to achieve success. A growth mindset, a concept popularized by psychologist Carol Dweck, is the belief that abilities and intelligence can be developed through dedication and hard work. This mindset fosters a love of learning, resilience in the face of challenges, and a passion for self-improvement.

Throughout this book, you'll learn how to cultivate a growth mindset, overcome limiting beliefs, and harness the power of positive thinking. By shifting your mindset, you'll be better equipped to tackle obstacles, seize opportunities, and realize your full potential.

Setting Intentions

Before diving into the strategies and exercises, it's important to set your intentions for this journey. What do you hope to achieve? What areas of your life do you want to improve?

Take a moment to reflect on your goals and write them down. Setting clear, intentional goals will give you direction and motivation as you work through the chapters.

Consider the following questions as you set your intentions:

- What are my top three goals for personal growth?
- Why are these goals important to me?
- How will achieving these goals impact my life?

By clearly defining your intentions, you'll create a roadmap that guides you through the process of personal development.

Commitment to Growth

Personal growth is a lifelong journey. It's not about reaching a final destination but continually striving to become the best version of yourself. This requires a commitment to growth, a dedication to learning, and a willingness to adapt and evolve. As you read this book and implement the strategies, keep in mind that growth takes time and effort. Be patient with yourself, celebrate your progress, and stay committed to your journey.

Your commitment to growth will be tested. There will be times when you feel discouraged, overwhelmed, or uncertain. In those moments, remind yourself of your intentions and the reasons behind your goals. Lean on the support of others, seek out resources, and stay focused on your vision. With perseverance and determination, you can overcome any obstacle and elevate your potential.

The Framework for Success

Holistic Approach

Elevating your potential requires a holistic approach that considers all aspects of your life. Personal growth is not confined to one area; it encompasses your mental, emotional, physical, and spiritual well-being. Throughout this book, you'll explore strategies that address each of these dimensions, ensuring a balanced and comprehensive approach to self-improvement.

- **Mental Well-being**: Developing a positive mindset, enhancing your intellectual capabilities, and fostering a love of learning.
- **Emotional Well-being**: Building emotional intelligence, managing stress, and cultivating resilience.
- **Physical Well-being**: Prioritizing health, fitness, and overall physical vitality.
- **Spiritual Well-being**: Connecting with your inner self, finding purpose, and aligning with your values.

By addressing these interconnected aspects of your life, you'll create a strong foundation for sustainable growth and success.

Practical and Actionable Strategies

This book is designed to be practical and actionable. Each chapter includes exercises, reflections, and real-life examples to help you apply the concepts to your own life. These strategies are grounded in research and proven methods, providing you with effective tools to elevate your potential.

- **Exercises**: Hands-on activities that encourage self-reflection, skill development, and practical application.
- **Reflections**: Thought-provoking questions that deepen your understanding and promote self-awareness.
- **Examples**: Real-life stories and case studies that illustrate key principles and offer inspiration.

As you work through the chapters, take the time to engage with these exercises and reflections. The more you actively participate, the more you'll gain from this journey.

The Power of Community

Building a Support System

Personal growth is not a solitary endeavor. Building a supportive community can significantly enhance your journey. Surrounding yourself with positive influences, mentors, and like-minded individuals provides encouragement, accountability, and diverse perspectives. In this book, you'll learn how to create and nurture a support system that empowers you to reach your goals.

- **Positive Influences**: Identifying and connecting with people who inspire and uplift you.

- **Mentorship**: Seeking guidance and wisdom from those who have walked a similar path.
- **Like-minded Individuals**: Engaging with a community that shares your values and aspirations.

Your support system can offer valuable insights, provide motivation during challenging times, and celebrate your successes alongside you.

Sharing Your Journey

As you progress on your journey, consider sharing your experiences with others. By openly discussing your challenges, successes, and learnings, you contribute to a culture of growth and support. Sharing your journey can also inspire and motivate others to embark on their own path of personal development.

- **Storytelling**: Sharing your personal stories and experiences to inspire and connect with others.
- **Accountability Partners**: Partnering with someone to mutually support and hold each other accountable.
- **Community Engagement**: Participating in groups, forums, or events focused on personal growth and development.

Together, we can create a ripple effect of positive change, fostering a community of individuals committed to elevating their potential.

Final Thoughts

As you embark on this journey of personal growth and success, remember that the power to elevate your potential lies within you. This book is your guide, providing the knowledge, tools, and inspiration needed to unlock that power. Take each step with intention, embrace the challenges, and celebrate your progress.

Your potential is limitless. With dedication, perseverance, and a commitment to growth, you can achieve extraordinary things. Welcome to the journey of elevating your potential—let's begin.

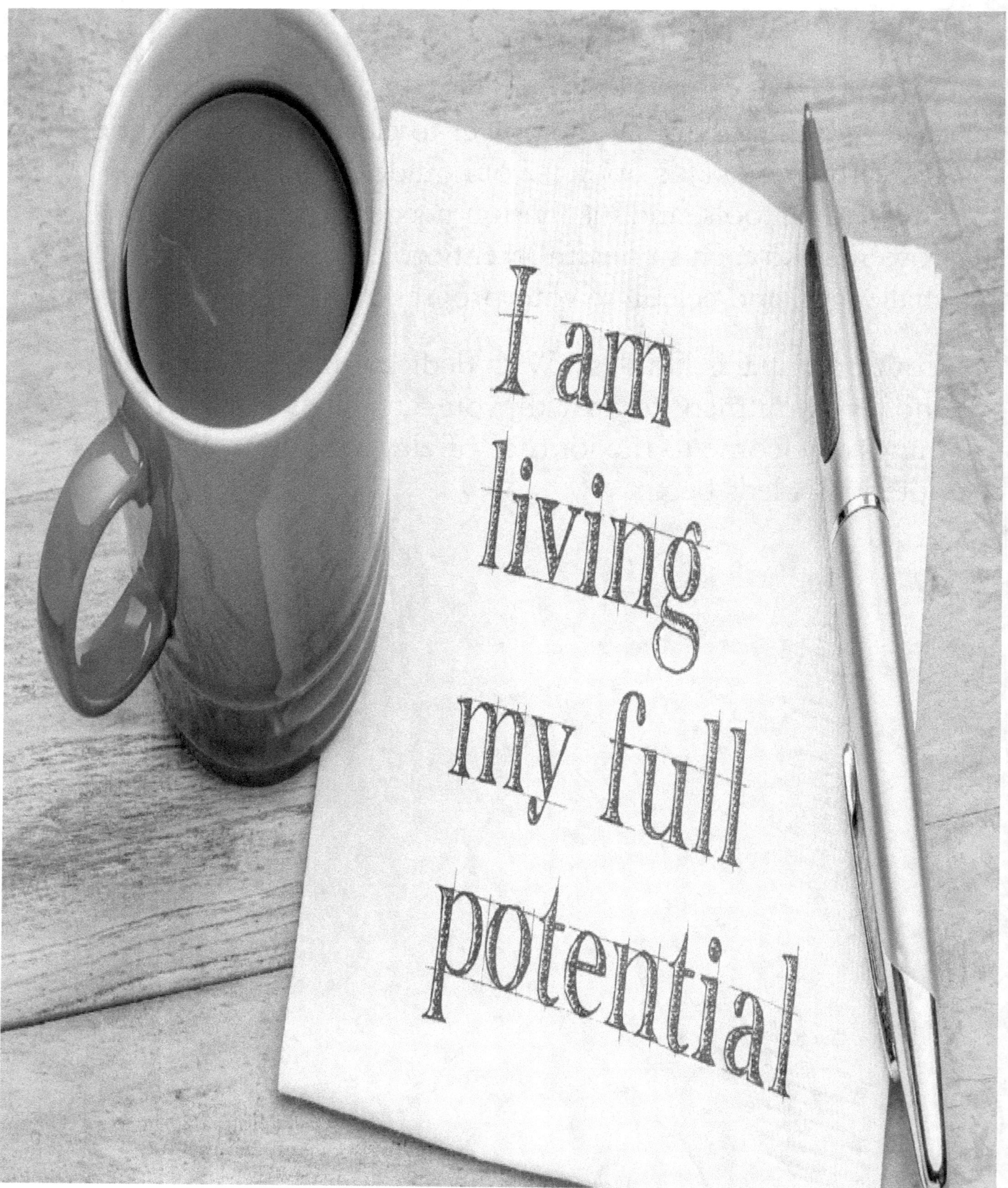
I am
living
my full
potential

Chapter 1: Understanding Potential

Introduction

What does it mean to have potential? How do you recognize it within yourself, and why is it so important to unlock it? In this chapter, we will explore these questions in depth, setting the foundation for your journey of personal growth and success.

Definition of Potential

Potential is the inherent ability or capacity for growth, development, or coming into being. It's the possibility that exists within each of us to achieve greatness, to rise above our current state, and to reach new heights. Understanding your potential means recognizing that you have untapped abilities and strengths waiting to be discovered and nurtured.

Illustrative Anecdote:

Imagine a seed. At first glance, it may seem small and insignificant. But within that seed lies the potential to become a towering tree. Similarly, within you lies the potential to grow and achieve great things. Just as the seed requires the right conditions to flourish, you too need the right mindset and tools to unlock your potential.

Recognizing Your Potential

Recognizing your potential begins with self-awareness. It's about taking an honest look at yourself—your strengths, weaknesses, passions, and dreams. Here are some steps to help you identify your potential:

1. **Assess Your Strengths and Weaknesses:**
   - Start by listing your strengths and weaknesses. This exercise helps you understand what you're naturally good at and areas where you may need improvement.
   - Strengths could include qualities like creativity, empathy, or problem-solving skills.
   - Weaknesses might be procrastination, impatience, or lack of focus.
2. **Identify Your Passions and Interests:**
   - What activities make you lose track of time? What topics do you enjoy learning about? These interests can point you toward your potential.
   - Reflect on hobbies, subjects, or activities that excite you and bring you joy.
3. **Seek Feedback from Others:**
   - Sometimes, others can see our potential more clearly than we can. Ask friends, family, or colleagues for their insights about your strengths and areas for growth.

- ○ Questions to ask might include: "What do you think I'm good at?" or "In what areas do you see me excelling?"
4. **Reflect on Past Successes:**
   - ○ Think about your past achievements. What skills or qualities helped you succeed? These can be indicators of your potential.
   - ○ Consider personal, academic, or professional accomplishments that made you proud.

Example:

Jane always enjoyed helping her friends resolve conflicts. She realized her potential as a mediator and pursued a career in conflict resolution. By recognizing her natural abilities and interests, Jane found a fulfilling and successful career path.

Detailed Case Study:

Case Study: John's Journey to Self-Discovery

John, a software developer, felt unfulfilled in his job despite his technical skills. He decided to explore his potential further. He listed his strengths as problem-solving and analytical thinking, and his weaknesses as poor communication and lack of creativity. John's passion lay in helping others and simplifying complex problems. After receiving feedback from his colleagues and reflecting on past projects, John realized his potential in teaching and mentoring. He started a blog to share his knowledge and eventually became a highly respected mentor in the tech community.

Importance of Unlocking Potential

Unlocking your potential is crucial for several reasons. It leads to personal fulfillment, drives success, and inspires others.

1. **Personal Fulfillment:**
   - Living up to your potential brings a deep sense of satisfaction. It means living a life true to your values and passions.
   - When you tap into your true abilities and pursue what you're passionate about, you experience a sense of satisfaction and purpose.
2. **Professional Success:**
   - When you harness your potential, you perform better in your career. Your unique strengths become your competitive advantage.
   - Recognizing and leveraging your strengths can propel you toward your goals more effectively.
3. **Inspiration to Others:**
   - By realizing your potential, you set an example for those around you, motivating them to pursue their own growth.
   - Your journey to unlocking your potential can inspire those around you.

Example:

Consider a teacher who discovers her potential in innovative teaching methods. Her unique approach not only benefits her students but also inspires fellow educators to explore new ways of teaching.

Practical Exercise: Discover Your Potential

To help you start recognizing your potential, try this practical exercise:

1. **Self-Reflection:**
   - Spend 15-30 minutes in a quiet space, reflecting on the following questions:
     - What are my top three strengths?
     - What activities make me feel most fulfilled?
     - When have I felt the most successful or proud of myself?
2. **Feedback from Others:**
   - Reach out to three people who know you well (friends, family, colleagues) and ask them:
     - What do you see as my greatest strengths?
     - In what areas do you think I have the most potential?
3. **Review and Plan:**

- Review your reflections and the feedback you received. Identify common themes and areas where you can focus your efforts to unlock your potential.

4. **Strengths Inventory:**
   - Create a comprehensive list of your strengths. Include skills, qualities, and talents. Write down specific examples of how you have demonstrated these strengths in the past.

5. **Passion Map:**
   - Draw a map of your interests and passions. Connect activities, subjects, and causes that excite you. Look for patterns and areas where your passions intersect with your strengths.

Reflection Questions

1. **Self-Reflection:**
   - What are my top three strengths?
   - What activities make me feel most fulfilled?
   - When have I felt the most successful or proud of myself?

2. **Feedback from Others:**
   - What do my friends, family, or colleagues see as my greatest strengths?
   - In what areas do they think I have the most potential?

3. **Action Plan:**
   - Based on your reflections and feedback, what are three specific actions you can take to start unlocking your potential?
4. **Strengths Inventory:**
   - How have I demonstrated my strengths in the past? Provide specific examples.
   - Which of my strengths do I enjoy using the most?
5. **Passion Map:**
   - What patterns do I see in my passions and interests?
   - How can I combine my passions with my strengths to pursue meaningful goals?

In-Depth Analysis: The Role of Environment

Your environment plays a significant role in unlocking your potential. A supportive and stimulating environment can nurture your growth, while a toxic or limiting environment can stifle it. Consider the following factors:

1. **Positive Influences:**
   - Surround yourself with people who encourage and support your growth. Seek mentors, join communities, and build relationships with individuals who inspire you.
2. **Learning Opportunities:**

- ○ Create an environment rich in learning opportunities. This could include reading books, attending workshops, or taking online courses related to your interests and goals.

3. **Physical Space:**
   - ○ Your physical space affects your productivity and creativity. Organize your workspace to minimize distractions and create an atmosphere conducive to focus and innovation.

4. **Mindful Consumption:**
   - ○ Be mindful of the information and media you consume. Choose content that motivates and educates you rather than distracts or discourages you.

Example:

Sarah, an aspiring writer, struggled to find her voice amidst the noise of daily life. She decided to create a dedicated writing space in her home, filled with inspirational books and minimal distractions. She also joined a local writers' group for support and feedback. This supportive environment allowed Sarah to unlock her potential and complete her first novel.

Expanded Practical Exercise: Environment Audit

Conduct an audit of your current environment to identify areas for improvement. This exercise will help you create a supportive and stimulating environment that nurtures your potential.

1. **Identify Positive Influences:**
   - List the people in your life who inspire and support you. Plan to spend more time with them and seek their guidance.
2. **Create Learning Opportunities:**
   - Identify resources such as books, courses, and workshops that align with your interests and goals. Schedule time to engage with these resources regularly.
3. **Optimize Your Physical Space:**
   - Evaluate your workspace. Remove clutter, add inspirational elements, and ensure it is conducive to focus and creativity.
4. **Mindful Media Consumption:**
   - Track the media and information you consume daily. Identify sources that motivate and educate you. Reduce exposure to content that distracts or discourages you.
5. **Action Plan:**
   - Based on your audit, create an action plan to enhance your environment. Set specific goals, such as organizing your workspace, joining a community, or limiting social media use.

Expanded Reflection Questions

1. **Self-Reflection:**
   - What changes can I make to my environment to better support my growth?
   - How can I increase my exposure to positive influences and learning opportunities?
2. **Feedback from Others:**
   - What do my friends, family, or colleagues suggest as improvements for my environment?
   - How can I involve them in creating a supportive environment?
3. **Action Plan:**
   - What are three specific actions I can take to optimize my physical space for productivity and creativity?
   - How can I ensure I consume media that motivates and educates me?
4. **Environment Audit:**
   - Who are the positive influences in my life, and how can I spend more time with them?
   - What learning opportunities are available to me, and how can I incorporate them into my routine?

Conclusion

Understanding and recognizing your potential is the first step in your journey toward personal growth and success. By assessing your strengths, identifying your passions, seeking feedback, and reflecting on your achievements, you can uncover the vast possibilities within you. Additionally, by optimizing your environment, you can create the conditions necessary for your growth. In the next chapter, we will delve into the power of mindset and motivation, crucial elements in unlocking your potential and driving your success.

"Failure is an opportunity to grow"
GROWTH MINDSET
"I can learn to do anything I want"
"Challenges help me to grow"
"My effort and attitude determine my abilities"
"Feedback is constructive"
"I am inspired by the success of others"
"I like to try new things"
"Failure is the limit of my abilities"
FIXED MINDSET
"I'm either good at it or I'm not"
"My abilities are unchanging"
"I don't like to be challenged"
"I can either do it, or I can't"
"My potential is predetermined"
"When I'm frustrated, I give up"
"Feedback and criticism are personal
"I stick to what I know"

Chapter 2: Mindset and Motivation

Growth vs. Fixed Mindset

One of the most critical aspects of personal development is understanding the difference between a growth mindset and a fixed mindset. The concept, popularized by psychologist Carol Dweck, highlights two fundamental attitudes towards learning and intelligence.

A **fixed mindset** is the belief that abilities and intelligence are static traits that cannot be significantly developed. People with a fixed mindset often avoid challenges, give up easily when faced with obstacles, see effort as fruitless, ignore useful feedback, and feel threatened by the success of others. This mindset can severely limit personal growth and achievement.

On the other hand, a **growth mindset** is the belief that abilities and intelligence can be developed through dedication, effort, and learning. Individuals with a growth mindset embrace challenges, persist through setbacks, see effort as the path to mastery, learn from criticism, and find inspiration in the success of others. This mindset fosters a love for learning and a resilience that is essential for great accomplishment.

Shifting from Fixed to Growth Mindset

- **Awareness**: The first step is to become aware of your mindset. Reflect on your reactions to challenges and feedback. Do you see them as opportunities to learn or threats to your competence?
- **Challenge Negative Thoughts**: When you catch yourself thinking in a fixed mindset way, challenge those thoughts. Replace "I can't do this" with "I can't do this yet."
- **Embrace Challenges**: Start seeing challenges as opportunities to grow rather than threats to your self-esteem. Every challenge you face is a chance to learn and improve.
- **Learn from Criticism**: Instead of getting defensive when receiving feedback, see it as a valuable source of information that can help you improve.
- **Celebrate Effort**: Focus on the effort you put in rather than the outcome. Recognize that effort leads to growth and improvement.

Techniques for Staying Motivated

Motivation is the driving force behind our actions. It's what keeps us going, even when the going gets tough. However, maintaining motivation can be challenging. Here are some techniques to help you stay motivated:

1. Set Clear Goals

- Having clear, specific goals gives you a direction and purpose. Break your long-term goals into smaller, manageable tasks. This makes them less overwhelming and provides a sense of accomplishment as you complete each one.

2. Find Your 'Why'

- Understanding the deeper reasons behind your goals can provide powerful motivation. Ask yourself why your goals are important to you. What will achieving them bring to your life? Keeping your 'why' in mind can fuel your perseverance.

3. Visualize Success

- Visualization is a powerful tool. Spend a few minutes each day visualizing yourself achieving your goals. Imagine the feelings of success, pride, and joy. This can boost your motivation and make your goals feel more attainable.

4. Create a Routine

- Consistency is key to maintaining motivation. Establish a daily or weekly routine that includes time dedicated to working on your goals. A routine helps build discipline and makes progress a habit.

5. Track Your Progress

- Keep a journal or use an app to track your progress. Seeing how far you've come can be incredibly motivating. Celebrate your achievements, no matter how small, to keep your spirits high.

6. Stay Positive

- Positive thinking can significantly impact your motivation. Surround yourself with positivity—positive people, positive affirmations, and positive media. When faced with setbacks, focus on what you can learn and how you can improve.

7. Reward Yourself

- Rewarding yourself for reaching milestones can keep you motivated. Treat yourself to something you enjoy when you achieve a goal. This creates a positive reinforcement loop that encourages continued effort.

8. Stay Accountable

- Share your goals with a friend, family member, or mentor. Having someone to check in with can provide accountability and support. They can offer encouragement and help you stay on track.

Overcoming Self-Doubt

Self-doubt can be a significant barrier to motivation and growth. It can make you question your abilities and hesitate to take action. Here are some strategies to overcome self-doubt:

1. Acknowledge Your Feelings

- It's essential to recognize and acknowledge your self-doubt rather than suppressing it. Accepting that you feel uncertain is the first step toward overcoming it.

2. Reframe Negative Thoughts

- Challenge negative self-talk by reframing it. Instead of thinking, "I'm not good enough," try "I am capable of learning and improving."

3. Focus on Your Strengths

- Remind yourself of your strengths and past successes. Reflect on the skills and qualities that have helped you achieve your goals before.

4. Take Small Steps

- Break your goals into smaller, achievable steps. Completing these small tasks can build your confidence and reduce feelings of self-doubt.

-

5. Seek Support

- Talk to someone you trust about your self-doubt. They can offer a different perspective and provide reassurance. Sometimes, just voicing your concerns can make them feel more manageable.

6. Practice Self-Compassion

- Be kind to yourself. Treat yourself with the same compassion and understanding you would offer a friend. Remember that everyone experiences self-doubt at times.

7. Keep Learning

- Self-doubt often stems from a fear of the unknown. Continuously learning and gaining new knowledge can boost your confidence and reduce uncertainty.

Practical Exercises and Reflection Questions

Exercise 1: Mindset Reflection

1. Reflect on a recent challenge you faced. How did you approach it? Did you have a fixed or growth mindset?
2. Write down three examples of fixed mindset thoughts you've had recently. Rewrite them as growth mindset thoughts.

Exercise 2: Motivation Journal

1. Set a specific goal for the next month. Break it down into weekly tasks.
2. Write down your 'why' for this goal. Why is it important to you?
3. Spend a few minutes each day visualizing yourself achieving this goal. Write about your experience and feelings in your journal.

Exercise 3: Overcoming Self-Doubt

1. Identify a situation where you experienced self-doubt. How did it affect your actions?
2. Write a letter to yourself from the perspective of a supportive friend. What encouraging words would they offer you?
3. List three strengths or past successes that can help you overcome your current self-doubt.

Reflection Questions

1. How do you currently view challenges and feedback? What steps can you take to shift towards a growth mindset?
2. What are your primary sources of motivation? How can you incorporate them into your daily routine?
3. In what areas of your life do you experience the most self-doubt? What strategies can you use to overcome it?

By applying these techniques and completing these exercises, you'll develop a stronger mindset and maintain the motivation needed to achieve your goals.

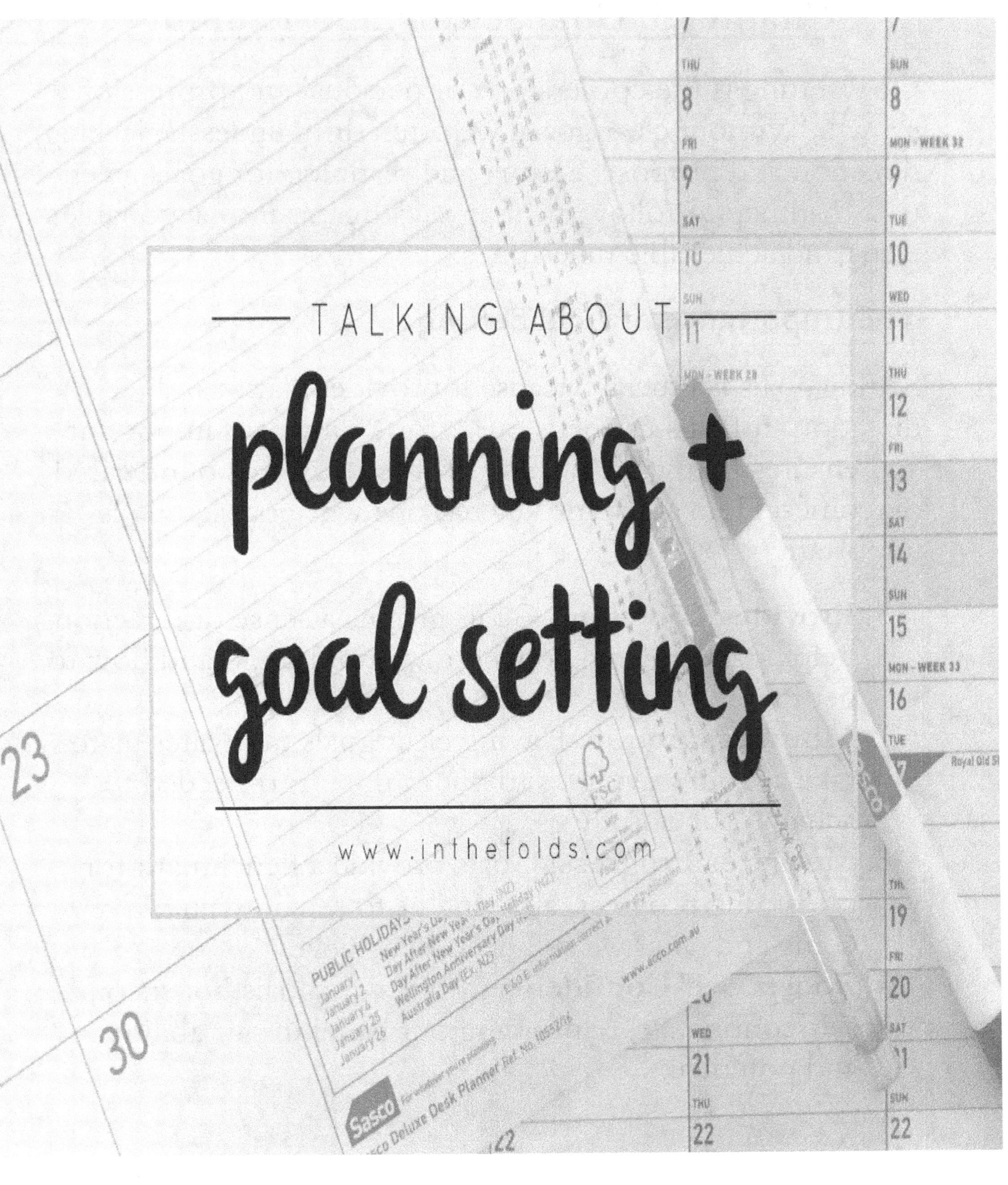

— TALKING ABOUT —
planning +
goal setting
www.inthefolds.com

Chapter 3: Goal Setting and Planning

Goal setting is the cornerstone of personal and professional growth. Without clear goals, we often drift aimlessly, lacking direction and purpose. Setting and planning for goals gives us a roadmap to follow, turning our dreams into actionable steps and achievable milestones.

The Importance of Goal Setting

Setting goals is crucial because it provides clarity and direction. It helps us focus our efforts on what's important and ensures that we're making progress towards our desired outcomes. Here are some key reasons why goal setting is important:

1. **Provides Direction**: Goals give us a sense of direction, helping us understand where we want to go and how to get there.
2. **Motivates Action**: Having clear goals motivates us to take action, driving us to put in the effort needed to achieve our objectives.
3. **Measures Progress**: Goals provide a benchmark for measuring progress, allowing us to see how far we've come and what we still need to achieve.
4. **Boosts Self-Confidence**: Achieving goals boosts our self-confidence, reinforcing our belief in our abilities and potential.

The SMART Framework

One of the most effective ways to set goals is by using the SMART framework. SMART goals are:

1. **Specific**: Clearly define what you want to achieve. The more specific your goal, the easier it is to understand and pursue.
    - Example: "I want to lose weight" vs. "I want to lose 10 pounds in 3 months by exercising and eating healthily."
2. **Measurable**: Ensure your goal is measurable so you can track your progress and know when you've achieved it.
    - Example: "I want to save money" vs. "I want to save $5,000 by the end of the year."
3. **Achievable**: Set realistic goals that are within your reach, considering your current abilities and resources.
    - Example: "I want to run a marathon next month" (if you've never run before) vs. "I want to run a 5K in three months."
4. **Relevant**: Ensure your goals align with your broader life objectives and values.
    - Example: "I want to learn French" (if you plan to move to France) vs. "I want to learn French" (without any context).
5. **Time-bound**: Set a deadline for your goal to create a sense of urgency and help you stay focused.

- Example: "I want to read more books" vs. "I want to read 12 books by the end of the year."

Creating Action Plans

Once you've set your SMART goals, the next step is to create a detailed action plan. This involves breaking down your goals into smaller, manageable tasks and setting timelines for each. Here's how you can create an effective action plan:

1. **Identify Key Steps**: Break your goal down into smaller steps that are necessary to achieve it.
   - Example: For the goal "I want to lose 10 pounds in 3 months," key steps might include creating a workout schedule, planning healthy meals, and tracking progress.
2. **Set Deadlines**: Assign deadlines to each step to ensure you stay on track and make consistent progress.
   - Example: "Join a gym by the end of the week," "Plan meals for the next week by Sunday."
3. **Prioritize Tasks**: Determine which tasks are most important and tackle them first. Prioritizing helps you focus on what will have the most significant impact.
   - Example: Prioritizing meal planning and regular exercise over less impactful activities.
4. **Track Progress**: Regularly review your progress and adjust your plan as needed. Tracking helps you stay accountable and make necessary adjustments.

- Example: Keeping a journal or using an app to log workouts and meals.

Overcoming Common Challenges

Achieving your goals often involves overcoming obstacles and challenges. Here are some common challenges and strategies to address them:

1. **Lack of Motivation**: Staying motivated can be challenging, especially for long-term goals.
   - **Solution**: Break your goal into smaller milestones and celebrate each achievement. Surround yourself with supportive people who encourage and motivate you.
2. **Procrastination**: Putting off tasks can hinder progress and cause stress.
   - **Solution**: Use techniques like the Pomodoro Technique (working in focused intervals) and eliminate distractions to stay on track.
3. **Fear of Failure**: The fear of not achieving your goals can be paralyzing.
   - **Solution**: Embrace failure as a learning opportunity. Reflect on what went wrong and use it to improve your approach.
4. **Lack of Resources**: Sometimes, we may not have the resources needed to achieve our goals.

- **Solution**: Identify alternative resources or adjust your goals to be more realistic given your current situation.

Practical Exercise: Setting Your SMART Goals

To help you set and plan your goals, try this practical exercise:

1. **Define Your Goal**: Write down a goal you want to achieve. Make sure it's specific, measurable, achievable, relevant, and time-bound.
   - Example: "I want to improve my public speaking skills by attending a weekly Toastmasters meeting for the next 6 months."
2. **Break It Down**: Identify the key steps needed to achieve your goal and assign deadlines to each.
   - Example:
     - Research local Toastmasters clubs (by end of week).
     - Attend the first meeting (by next week).
     - Prepare and deliver a speech (within the first month).
3. **Track Progress**: Create a system to track your progress. This could be a journal, an app, or a calendar.
   - Example: Use a journal to reflect on each meeting and track improvements in your speaking skills.
4. **Review and Adjust**: Regularly review your progress and make adjustments as needed.

- o Example: If you're struggling with certain aspects of public speaking, seek feedback from peers and focus on those areas in subsequent meetings.

Reflection Questions

1. What are some of your long-term goals, and why are they important to you?
2. How can you break down a large goal into smaller, manageable tasks?
3. What obstacles have you encountered when setting goals in the past, and how did you overcome them?
4. How do you plan to track your progress and stay motivated while working towards your goals?
5. What steps will you take to ensure your goals align with your broader life objectives and values?

❖ *(this image is taken from betterUp)*

Chapter 4: Building Positive Habits

The Power of Habit

Habits shape our lives in profound ways. They are the building blocks of daily routines, driving our behaviors and decisions. A habit is a routine or practice performed regularly; it's an automatic response to specific situations or cues. When these habits are positive, they can lead to significant improvements in our lives. Conversely, negative habits can hold us back and hinder our progress.

Imagine waking up every morning and starting your day with a healthy breakfast, followed by a quick workout. This positive routine sets the tone for the day, boosting your energy levels and improving your mood. On the other hand, starting your day by hitting the snooze button multiple times and skipping breakfast can lead to a sluggish, unproductive day.

The power of habit lies in its consistency. By developing positive habits, you create a strong foundation for personal growth and success. The key is to understand how habits work and how to build and maintain them effectively.

How Habits Work: The Habit Loop

Habits operate through a simple neurological loop consisting of three elements: cue, routine, and reward.

1. **Cue**: The trigger that initiates the habit. It could be a time of day, an emotion, a specific place, or an action.
2. **Routine**: The behavior or action performed in response to the cue.
3. **Reward**: The positive outcome or feeling derived from the routine, reinforcing the habit loop.

For example, consider the habit of drinking a cup of coffee every morning.

- **Cue**: Waking up in the morning.
- **Routine**: Making and drinking a cup of coffee.
- **Reward**: Feeling awake and alert, ready to start the day.

Understanding this loop is crucial for developing new habits or changing existing ones. By identifying and modifying the elements of the loop, you can create positive habits that stick.

Steps to Build New Habits

1. **Start Small**

When building new habits, it's essential to start small. Overambitious goals can lead to burnout and discouragement. Instead, focus on one small change at a time. For instance, if you want to start exercising regularly, begin with a short 5-minute workout each day. Gradually increase the duration and intensity as the habit becomes ingrained.

2. Be Consistent

Consistency is key to habit formation. Choose a specific time or context for your new habit to ensure it becomes a regular part of your routine. Consistency reinforces the habit loop, making it easier for the behavior to become automatic. If you decide to meditate every evening, do it at the same time and place each day.

3. Use Triggers

Identify cues that will trigger your new habit. Triggers are essential because they remind you to perform the behavior. Pair your new habit with an existing one to create a strong trigger. For example, if you want to develop a habit of reading before bed, place your book on your pillow each morning so that it's ready when you go to bed.

4. Reward Yourself

Rewards reinforce habits by providing positive feedback. After completing your new habit, give yourself a small reward. This could be a treat, a moment of relaxation, or simply acknowledging your progress. Over time, the reward becomes associated with the routine, strengthening the habit loop.

5. Track Your Progress

Keeping track of your progress can be motivating and help you stay accountable. Use a habit tracker or journal to record each time you complete your new habit. Seeing your progress visually can reinforce your commitment and provide a sense of accomplishment.

6. Be Patient

Building new habits takes time. It's important to be patient with yourself and recognize that setbacks are a natural part of the process. If you miss a day or encounter difficulties, don't be too hard on yourself. Instead, focus on getting back on track and maintaining your commitment.

Maintaining Consistency

Maintaining consistency is crucial for long-term habit formation. Here are some strategies to help you stay consistent:

1. Set Realistic Goals

Set achievable goals that align with your current lifestyle and capabilities. Unrealistic expectations can lead to frustration and burnout. Start with small, manageable habits and gradually build up to more significant changes.

2. Create a Routine

Incorporate your new habit into your daily routine. Consistency is easier to achieve when the habit becomes a natural part of your day. For example, if you want to start journaling, do it every morning with your coffee or every evening before bed.

3. Find Accountability

Share your habit goals with a friend, family member, or accountability partner. Having someone to check in with can provide support, encouragement, and motivation. You can also join online communities or groups focused on similar goals.

4. Celebrate Milestones

Celebrate your progress and milestones along the way. Acknowledging your achievements, no matter how small, can boost your motivation and reinforce your commitment. Treat yourself to something special or simply take a moment to reflect on how far you've come.

5. Adjust as Needed

Be flexible and willing to adjust your approach if necessary. Life can be unpredictable, and sometimes, your routine may need to change. If you encounter obstacles, find alternative ways to maintain your habit. For example, if you can't go to the gym, do a home workout instead.

6. Stay Positive

Maintain a positive mindset and focus on the benefits of your new habit. Visualize the positive outcomes and how they contribute to your overall well-being and success. Positive reinforcement can help you stay motivated and committed to your habit.

Practical Exercises and Reflection Questions

Exercise 1: Identify Your Triggers

Take some time to identify potential triggers for a new habit you want to build. Reflect on your daily routine and find a specific cue that can remind you to perform the new habit. Write down the cue and how you will use it to trigger your habit.

Reflection Question: What existing routine or activity can I pair with my new habit to create a strong trigger?

Exercise 2: Create a Habit Tracker

Design a simple habit tracker to monitor your progress. Each day you complete your new habit, mark it on the tracker. This visual representation will help you stay accountable and motivated. Keep the tracker in a visible place where you can see it daily.

Reflection Question: How does tracking my progress visually impact my motivation and commitment to my new habit?

Exercise 3: Plan Your Rewards

Think about small rewards you can give yourself after completing your new habit. Write down a list of rewards that will motivate you and provide positive reinforcement. Make sure the rewards are meaningful and enjoyable.

Reflection Question: What rewards will genuinely motivate me to maintain my new habit consistently?

Exercise 4: Set Realistic Goals

Set a specific, achievable goal for your new habit. Break it down into smaller, manageable steps. Write down your goal and the steps you will take to achieve it. Review and adjust your goals as needed to ensure they remain realistic.

Reflection Question: How can I break down my new habit into smaller, manageable steps to ensure success?

Exercise 5: Find an Accountability Partner

Identify someone who can support and hold you accountable for your new habit. Share your goals and progress with them regularly. Schedule check-ins to discuss your achievements and challenges.

Reflection Question: Who can I rely on to provide support and accountability as I work on building my new habit?

Exercise 6: Reflect on Your Progress

Set aside time each week to reflect on your progress. Review your habit tracker, celebrate your achievements, and identify any challenges you encountered. Adjust your approach if necessary and recommit to your goals.

Reflection Question: What challenges did I face this week, and how can I overcome them to maintain my new habit?

By understanding the power of habits and implementing these strategies, you can build positive habits that support your personal growth and success. Remember, the key to lasting change lies in consistency, patience, and a positive mindset. Embrace the journey of habit formation and enjoy the transformative impact it will have on your life.

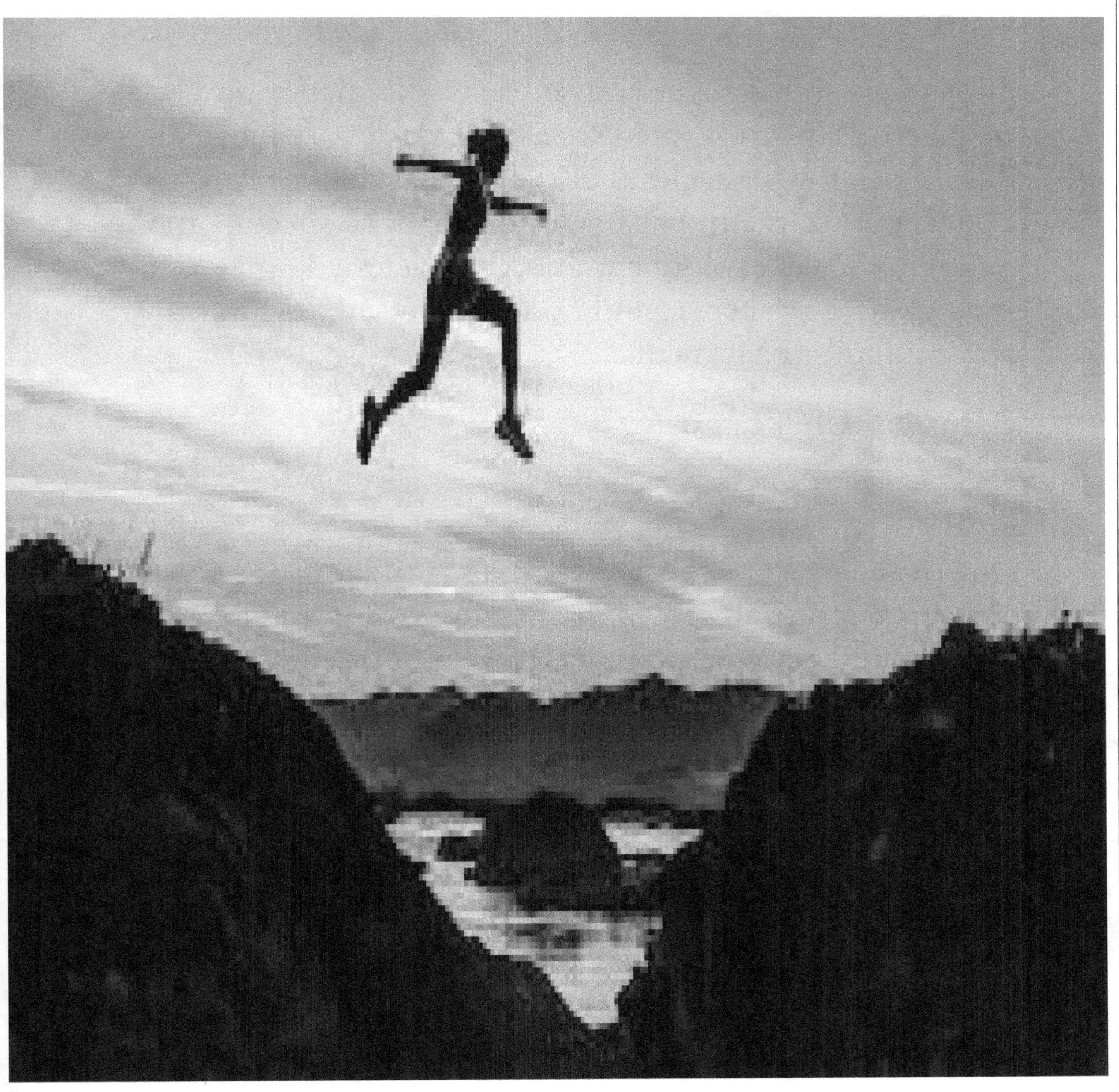

Chapter 5: Overcoming Obstacles

Introduction

Life is full of challenges and setbacks. No matter how well we plan or how motivated we are, obstacles are inevitable. But it's not the obstacles themselves that define us; it's how we respond to them that shapes our path to success. In this chapter, we will explore common obstacles you may face, strategies for resilience, and how to turn setbacks into opportunities for growth.

Common Challenges

Fear of Failure

One of the most pervasive obstacles is the fear of failure. This fear can paralyze you, preventing you from taking risks or pursuing your goals. However, it's important to remember that failure is not the end—it's a stepping stone to success. Every failure teaches you something valuable and brings you one step closer to your goals.

Overcoming Fear of Failure:

1. **Reframe Failure:** See failure as a learning opportunity rather than a setback. Each failure provides insights that can help you improve.
2. **Small Steps:** Break your goals into smaller, manageable tasks. Achieving these smaller tasks builds confidence and reduces the fear of failure.

3. **Positive Visualization:** Visualize your success and the steps you need to take to get there. Positive visualization can boost your confidence and reduce fear.

Lack of Confidence

Confidence is key to overcoming obstacles. Without it, even minor challenges can seem insurmountable. Building confidence takes time and practice, but it's essential for personal growth.

Building Confidence:

1. **Self-Affirmations:** Use positive affirmations to reinforce your belief in yourself. Phrases like "I am capable" and "I can handle this" can boost your confidence.
2. **Celebrate Successes:** Take time to celebrate your achievements, no matter how small. Recognizing your successes reinforces your self-worth.
3. **Skill Development:** Continuously work on improving your skills. The more competent you become, the more confident you will feel.

External Criticism

Criticism from others can be discouraging. It's important to learn how to handle criticism constructively without letting it undermine your confidence.

Handling Criticism:

1. **Constructive Feedback:** Distinguish between constructive feedback and destructive criticism. Use constructive feedback to improve and ignore baseless criticism.
2. **Seek Supportive Voices:** Surround yourself with people who support and encourage you. Their positive reinforcement can help you stay focused on your goals.
3. **Internal Validation:** Learn to validate yourself. Your worth is not determined by others' opinions. Believe in your abilities and stay true to your path.

Strategies for Resilience

Resilience is the ability to bounce back from setbacks and keep moving forward. Developing resilience is crucial for overcoming obstacles and achieving long-term success.

Mindfulness and Stress Management

Stress can be a major obstacle. Practicing mindfulness and stress management techniques can help you stay calm and focused in the face of challenges.

Practicing Mindfulness:

1. **Breathing Exercises:** Simple breathing exercises can reduce stress and help you stay grounded. Try deep breathing or box breathing techniques.

2. **Meditation:** Regular meditation practice can improve your ability to handle stress and increase your overall sense of well-being.
3. **Mindful Awareness:** Pay attention to your thoughts and feelings without judgment. Recognize stress triggers and address them constructively.

Developing a Growth Mindset

A growth mindset is the belief that abilities and intelligence can be developed through effort and learning. Embracing a growth mindset can help you see obstacles as opportunities for growth.

Cultivating a Growth Mindset:

1. **Embrace Challenges:** See challenges as opportunities to learn and grow. Each challenge you overcome makes you stronger.
2. **Learn from Criticism:** Use criticism as feedback for improvement. A growth mindset values learning and growth over perfection.
3. **Persistence:** Keep pushing forward, even when things get tough. Persistence is key to overcoming obstacles and achieving success.

Building a Support Network

Having a strong support network can make a significant difference when facing obstacles. Surrounding yourself with supportive and positive people can provide the encouragement and assistance you need to overcome challenges.

Creating a Support Network:

1. **Seek Mentors:** Find mentors who can offer guidance and support based on their experiences.
2. **Build Relationships:** Cultivate relationships with friends, family, and colleagues who share your values and goals.
3. **Join Communities:** Engage in communities or groups that align with your interests and aspirations. Shared experiences can offer valuable insights and support.

Turning Setbacks into Opportunities

Every setback has the potential to become an opportunity for growth and development. The key is to maintain a positive outlook and be proactive in finding solutions.

Reassessing Goals

Setbacks can be an opportunity to reassess your goals and strategies. Sometimes, a change in direction can lead to even greater success.

Reevaluating Your Goals:

1. **Reflect:** Take time to reflect on your goals and the reasons behind them. Are they still aligned with your values and aspirations?
2. **Adjust Plans:** Be flexible and willing to adjust your plans if necessary. Adaptability is crucial for navigating obstacles.
3. **Set New Goals:** If needed, set new goals that better reflect your current situation and long-term vision.

Learning from Mistakes

Mistakes are a natural part of the learning process. Analyzing and learning from your mistakes can provide valuable lessons for future success.

Analyzing Mistakes:

1. **Identify the Cause:** Understand what led to the mistake. Was it a lack of information, a wrong approach, or external factors?
2. **Learn and Adapt:** Use the insights gained to improve your strategies and decision-making processes.
3. **Move Forward:** Let go of the guilt associated with mistakes. Focus on moving forward with the lessons learned.

Maintaining a positive attitude and staying motivated is essential for overcoming obstacles. Positivity fuels perseverance and resilience.

Staying Positive:

1. **Gratitude Practice:** Regularly practice gratitude. Focus on the positive aspects of your life and acknowledge your achievements.
2. **Positive Visualization:** Visualize your success and the positive outcomes you desire. Visualization can boost motivation and confidence.
3. **Self-Care:** Prioritize self-care to maintain your physical and mental well-being. A healthy mind and body are better equipped to handle challenges.

Practical Exercises and Reflection Questions

Practical Exercise 1: Reframing Failure

1. **Think of a Recent Failure:** Identify a recent situation where you feel you failed.
2. **Reframe the Failure:** Write down three positive things you learned from that experience.
3. **Plan for Improvement:** Outline steps you can take to avoid similar failures in the future.

Practical Exercise 2: Building Confidence

1. **Self-Affirmation List:** Create a list of ten positive affirmations about yourself. Read them aloud daily.
2. **Celebrate Small Wins:** Keep a journal where you write down one achievement or success each day, no matter how small.
3. **Skill Improvement Plan:** Identify one skill you want to improve. Create a plan with actionable steps and set a timeline for progress.

Reflection Questions

1. What is your biggest fear when it comes to pursuing your goals? How can you reframe this fear to see it as a learning opportunity?
2. Think about a time when external criticism affected you. How did you respond, and what could you have done differently to handle it constructively?
3. Describe a recent setback you experienced. What did you learn from it, and how can you use this knowledge to move forward positively?
4. Who are the people in your life that provide the most support and encouragement? How can you strengthen these relationships further?
5. Reflect on a time when you overcame a significant obstacle. What strategies did you use, and how can you apply those strategies to future challenges?

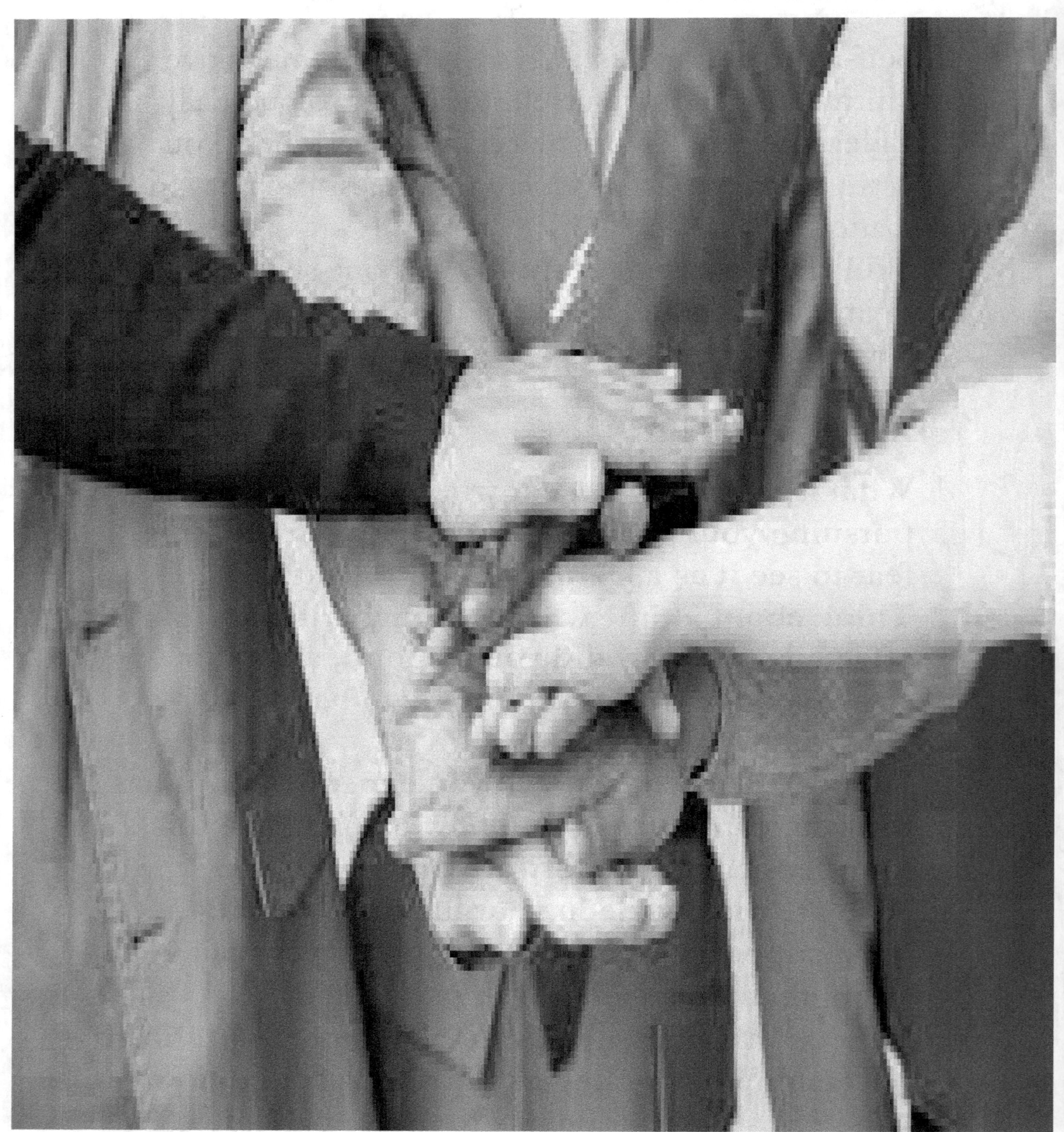

`Chapter 6: Leveraging Strengths and Skills

Introduction

Leveraging your strengths and skills is pivotal in achieving personal growth and success. Understanding what you naturally excel at, combined with a willingness to develop new capabilities, can significantly propel you towards your goals. This chapter will guide you through the process of identifying your strengths, developing new skills, and applying them effectively in various aspects of your life.

Identifying Strengths

Self-Assessment

The journey to leveraging your strengths begins with self-assessment. Knowing what you excel at naturally can provide a strong foundation for personal growth. Here are some steps to identify your strengths:

1. **Reflect on Past Successes**: Think about times when you felt particularly successful or proud of your accomplishments. What were you doing? What skills or qualities did you use?

   Example: Reflecting on her career, Jane realized that her most significant successes involved leading projects and solving complex problems. These moments made her feel energized and fulfilled.

2. **Personality Tests**: Tools like the Myers-Briggs Type Indicator (MBTI), StrengthsFinder, or VIA Character Strengths can provide insights into your natural preferences and strengths.

   Example: Tom discovered through the StrengthsFinder assessment that his top strengths were strategic thinking, relationship building, and influencing others. This knowledge helped him focus on roles that leveraged these strengths.

3. **Feedback from Others**: Sometimes, others see strengths in us that we might overlook. Ask friends, family, and colleagues for feedback on what they perceive to be your strongest qualities.

   Example: Sara's colleagues consistently praised her for her exceptional communication skills and her ability to mediate conflicts. This feedback helped her realize the value of her interpersonal skills.

4. **Journaling**: Keep a journal where you record your daily activities and note times when you felt particularly energized or accomplished. Patterns may emerge that highlight your strengths.

   Example: By journaling, Mark noticed that he felt most satisfied and productive when he was engaged in creative problem-solving and brainstorming sessions.

Real-Life Example

Consider Sarah, a project manager in a tech company. Through self-assessment, Sarah realized that her key strengths were organization, communication, and problem-solving. By focusing on these strengths, she was able to lead her team more effectively and deliver projects on time, even under tight deadlines. Her ability to organize tasks, communicate clearly, and solve problems quickly made her an invaluable asset to her team.

Deep Dive into Strengths

Understanding your strengths isn't just about listing them; it's about understanding how they manifest in different situations. For example, if one of your strengths is empathy, consider how it helps you in various aspects of your life—personal relationships, professional interactions, and even in community settings.

1. **Contextual Application**: Think about how your strengths show up in different contexts. Are you particularly good at resolving conflicts at work because of your empathy? Does your organizational skill help you manage family events efficiently?
2. **Strengths in Challenges**: Reflect on times when your strengths helped you overcome significant challenges. How did they aid you, and what was the outcome?
3. **Natural vs. Developed Strengths**: Identify which strengths come naturally to you and which ones you

have developed over time. Understanding this can help you focus on honing both types effectively.

Developing New Skills

While leveraging existing strengths is crucial, developing new skills can open up additional opportunities and help you adapt to changing circumstances. Here's how you can approach skill development:

1. **Identify Skill Gaps**: Determine which skills are necessary for your goals that you currently lack. This could involve technical skills, soft skills, or industry-specific knowledge.

   Example: Rachel, aiming to become a team leader, identified a gap in her leadership skills. She realized that to lead effectively, she needed to enhance her ability to delegate tasks and manage conflicts.

2. **Create a Learning Plan**: Set specific, achievable goals for learning new skills. This might include taking courses, reading books, attending workshops, or finding a mentor.

   Example: To develop his coding skills, James enrolled in an online programming course, set aside dedicated time each day for practice, and joined a local coding club to gain hands-on experience.

3. **Practice and Application**: The best way to solidify new skills is through practice. Seek opportunities to apply what you've learned in real-world scenarios.

   Example: After learning about project management techniques, Alice volunteered to manage a small project at work. This allowed her to apply her new skills and gain practical experience.

4. **Continuous Improvement**: Keep a growth mindset. Regularly seek feedback and be willing to make adjustments to improve further.

   Example: David adopted a continuous improvement approach by regularly seeking feedback from his peers and supervisors on his presentation skills. This iterative process helped him become a more effective communicator.

Real-Life Example

John, a marketing professional, wanted to move into a managerial role but lacked leadership skills. He enrolled in leadership courses, read extensively on management strategies, and sought mentorship from experienced leaders in his organization. Over time, John's efforts paid off, and he was promoted to a managerial position. His journey illustrates the importance of continuous learning and practical application in skill development.

Developing Soft Skills

Soft skills such as communication, empathy, and teamwork are often as important, if not more so, than technical skills. These skills enable you to interact effectively with others and navigate the social complexities of the workplace.

1. **Communication Skills**: Enhance your ability to convey ideas clearly and listen actively.

   Example: Maria attended workshops on effective communication and practiced active listening with her team, leading to better collaboration and fewer misunderstandings.

2. **Emotional Intelligence**: Develop your ability to understand and manage your own emotions and those of others.

   Example: By reading books on emotional intelligence and applying the principles in her daily interactions, Lisa improved her relationships both at work and in her personal life.

3. **Teamwork and Collaboration**: Foster a collaborative spirit and learn to work well in team settings.

   Example: Michael joined a volunteer group where he could practice teamwork skills in a low-stakes environment, which translated into better collaboration at his job.

Technical Skills

In many fields, technical skills are essential. Whether it's proficiency in software, understanding complex systems, or staying updated with industry-specific knowledge, technical skills can significantly enhance your professional capabilities.

1. **Stay Updated**: Regularly update your technical knowledge through courses, webinars, and industry publications.

   Example: Olivia, a software engineer, subscribed to several tech journals and attended industry conferences to stay abreast of the latest developments in her field.

2. **Hands-On Practice**: Practice your technical skills through real-world applications, side projects, or by contributing to open-source projects.

   Example: Ethan, aspiring to be a data scientist, worked on personal data projects and shared his findings on online forums, gaining practical experience and feedback.

3. **Certifications**: Obtain relevant certifications to validate your skills and enhance your credibility.

   Example: Emily pursued a project management certification, which not only improved her skills but also made her more attractive to potential employers.

Applying Strengths and Skills Effectively

To truly leverage your strengths and skills, you need to apply them strategically in your personal and professional life. Here are some tips:

1. **Align with Your Goals**: Ensure that the activities you focus on align with your long-term goals. Use your strengths to work towards these objectives.

   Example: Nathan's goal was to become a leading sales manager. He focused on honing his strengths in communication and relationship-building, which were directly aligned with his career aspirations.

2. **Seek Opportunities**: Look for situations where your strengths can shine. Volunteer for projects or roles that allow you to use your skills.

   Example: Rebecca, with a knack for event planning, volunteered to organize her company's annual conference. This opportunity allowed her to showcase her organizational and leadership skills.

3. **Collaborate with Others**: Complement your strengths by collaborating with others who have different skill sets. This synergy can lead to better outcomes.

   Example: Alex, a talented writer, partnered with a graphic designer to create compelling marketing materials. Their combined skills resulted in a highly effective campaign.

4. **Stay Adaptable**: Be open to new experiences and opportunities that may arise. Flexibility can help you apply your strengths in diverse situations.

   Example: Chloe, a finance professional, was open to taking on a temporary role in operations. This experience broadened her skill set and provided new insights into her organization.

Real-Life Example

Emma, a graphic designer, found that her creativity and attention to detail were her biggest strengths. She took on projects that allowed her to showcase these abilities, leading to high client satisfaction and an expanded portfolio. By consistently seeking opportunities that matched her strengths, Emma's career flourished. She also collaborated with marketing professionals to create comprehensive branding strategies, which enhanced her creative output and led to more successful projects.

Strength-Based Leadership

Leadership roles often require a diverse skill set. Leveraging your strengths can make you a more effective leader. Understand your leadership style and how your strengths can support your team.

1. **Identify Your Leadership Style**: Are you a transformational leader who inspires others, or a transactional leader who focuses on tasks and rewards?

   Example: Jason realized he was a transformational leader. He used his strength in inspiring others to motivate his team and drive innovation.

2. **Delegate Based on Strengths**: Recognize the strengths of your team members and delegate tasks that align with their abilities.

   Example: Laura identified that one team member excelled in data analysis, while another was great at client interactions. She delegated tasks accordingly, which improved team efficiency and morale.

3. **Empower Your Team**: Use your strengths to empower and develop your team members, fostering a supportive and productive environment.

   Example: Using her strength in coaching, Megan provided regular feedback and development opportunities for her team, leading to improved performance and job satisfaction.

Practical Exercises

Exercise 1: Strengths Inventory

1. List your top five strengths. Reflect on past experiences, feedback from others, and self-assessment tools.
2. For each strength, write down specific instances where you used this strength effectively.
3. Identify at least three ways you can use each strength more frequently in your daily life or work.

Exercise 2: Skill Development Plan

1. Identify two skills you want to develop that are important for your goals.
2. Research resources (courses, books, mentors) that can help you learn these skills.
3. Create a timeline with specific milestones for practicing and applying these skills.

Exercise 3: SWOT Analysis

1. Conduct a SWOT analysis (Strengths, Weaknesses, Opportunities, Threats) on yourself.
2. Identify how you can leverage your strengths to take advantage of opportunities and mitigate threats.
3. Develop a plan to address your weaknesses.

Exercise 4: Leadership Application

1. Reflect on your leadership style and identify your core strengths.
2. Create a plan to leverage these strengths to enhance your leadership effectiveness.
3. Implement strategies to delegate tasks based on team members' strengths.

Exercise 5: Strengths-Based Goal Setting

1. Set three personal or professional goals that align with your strengths.
2. Develop an action plan to achieve these goals, focusing on utilizing your strengths.
3. Monitor your progress and adjust your plan as needed.

Reflection Questions

1. What are your core strengths, and how do they align with your personal and professional goals?
2. How have you successfully applied your strengths in the past? Can you replicate those situations?
3. What new skills do you need to develop to reach your next level of growth? What steps will you take to acquire these skills?
4. How can you create more opportunities to leverage your strengths in your current environment?
5. In what ways can collaborating with others enhance your ability to apply your strengths effectively?

Conclusion

Leveraging your strengths and skills is a continuous journey of self-discovery and development. By understanding your unique abilities, developing new skills, and applying them effectively, you can achieve greater success and fulfillment in both your personal and professional life. Embrace this process with an open mind and a proactive attitude, and watch as you unlock your true potential.

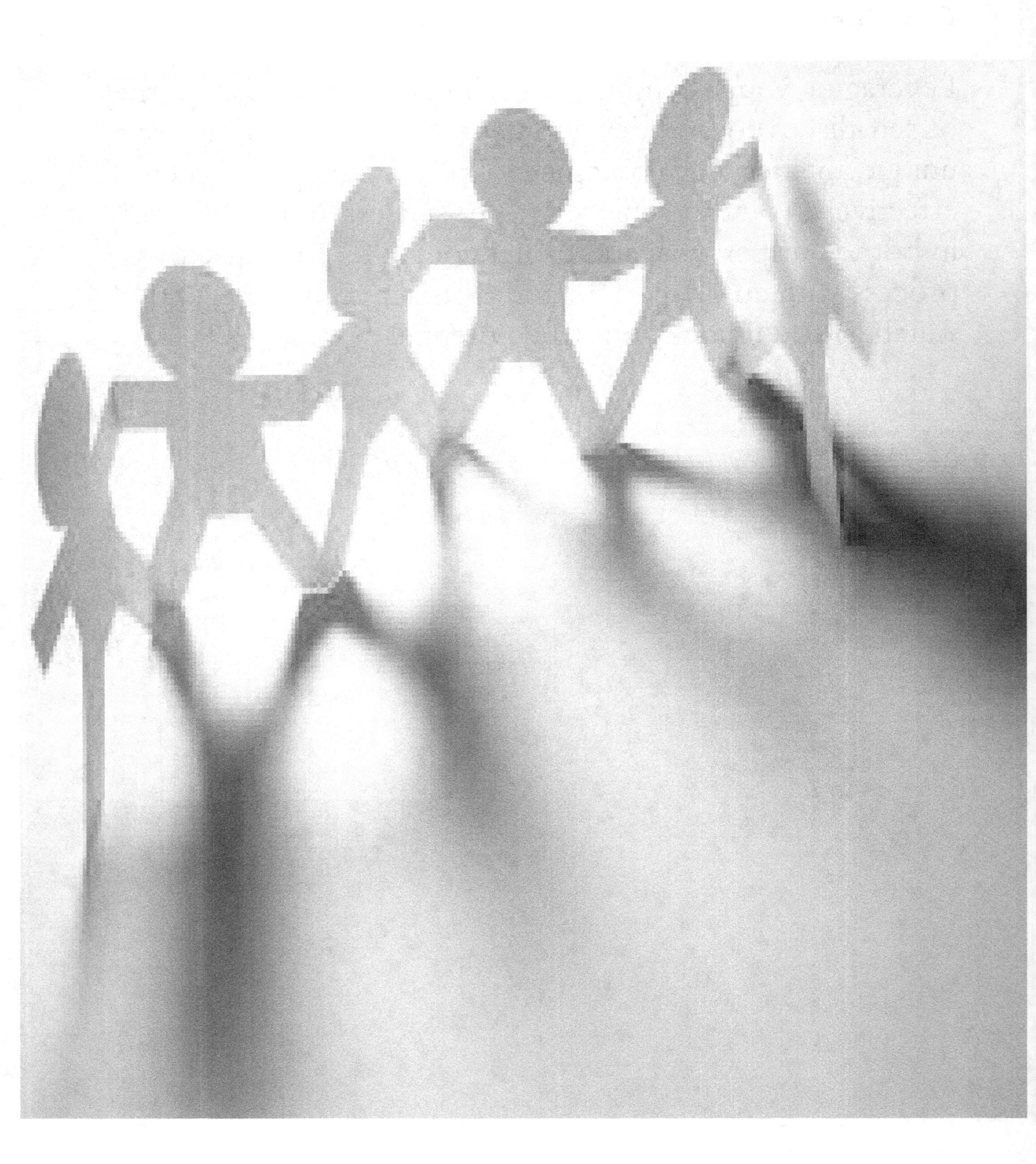

Chapter 7: Creating a Supportive Environment

Introduction: The Power of Your Environment

Imagine a seed trying to grow in rocky soil versus fertile, nutrient-rich soil. The environment makes all the difference. Similarly, your personal and professional growth is significantly influenced by the environment you create around yourself. A supportive environment can nurture your potential, helping you thrive and achieve your goals. This chapter will guide you on how to build such an environment, emphasizing the importance of positive influences, a strong support network, and managing negative elements.

The Role of Positive Influences

Positive influences are like the sun and rain for a growing plant—they provide the energy and nourishment needed for growth. Surrounding yourself with positive people and influences can boost your motivation, provide encouragement, and offer valuable perspectives.

1. **Identify Positive Influences**: Take note of the people who inspire and uplift you. These could be friends, family, mentors, or colleagues. What qualities do they possess that you admire? How do they contribute to your growth?
2. **Engage with Positive Media**: The media you consume also shapes your environment. Choose books,

podcasts, and social media that promote positivity and personal growth. Limit exposure to negative or toxic content that drains your energy.

3. **Practice Gratitude**: Cultivating an attitude of gratitude can transform your outlook. Regularly acknowledging and appreciating the positive aspects of your life can create a more supportive and uplifting environment.

Building a Strong Support Network

A strong support network is essential for navigating life's challenges and achieving your goals. These are the people who believe in you, support your endeavors, and stand by you during tough times.

1. **Nurture Relationships**: Invest time and effort into building and maintaining meaningful relationships. Show genuine interest in others, offer support when needed, and be there for them as they are for you.
2. **Seek Mentorship**: Having mentors can provide invaluable guidance and insights. Look for individuals who have achieved what you aspire to and seek their advice. Mentorship can accelerate your growth by helping you avoid common pitfalls and navigate challenges effectively.
3. **Join Communities**: Being part of a community with shared interests and goals can provide a sense of belonging and mutual support. Whether it's a professional group, hobby club, or online community,

engaging with like-minded individuals can foster growth and motivation.

Managing Negative Influences

Just as important as cultivating positive influences is managing and minimizing negative ones. Negative influences can drain your energy, lower your motivation, and hinder your progress.

1. **Identify Negative Influences**: Reflect on the people, situations, and habits that negatively impact you. These could be toxic relationships, unsupportive colleagues, or destructive habits. Recognizing these influences is the first step towards managing them.
2. **Set Boundaries**: Learn to set and maintain healthy boundaries. This might mean limiting time spent with negative individuals, avoiding certain situations, or saying no to commitments that don't align with your goals.
3. **Practice Self-Care**: Taking care of your mental, emotional, and physical well-being is crucial in managing negative influences. Regular self-care practices can help you stay resilient and maintain a positive outlook.

Creating a Positive Physical Environment

Your physical surroundings also play a crucial role in your well-being and productivity. A cluttered or chaotic environment can lead to stress and distraction, while an organized and inspiring space can boost your motivation and focus.

1. **Declutter and Organize**: Regularly declutter your space and organize it in a way that promotes efficiency and calm. A clean and orderly environment can reduce stress and improve your ability to concentrate.
2. **Personalize Your Space**: Add elements to your environment that inspire and motivate you. This could be inspirational quotes, photos of loved ones, or items related to your goals and passions.
3. **Create a Productive Atmosphere**: Ensure your environment is conducive to productivity. This might involve setting up a dedicated workspace, minimizing distractions, and having the necessary tools and resources readily available.

Practical Exercises and Reflection Questions

To help you create a supportive environment, try these exercises and reflect on the following questions:

1. **Positive Influence Inventory**: Make a list of the people who have a positive impact on your life. Write down specific ways they support and inspire you. How can you spend more time with these individuals or learn from them?
2. **Media Audit**: Assess the media you consume daily. Identify any sources that consistently bring negativity

into your life. Replace them with positive, uplifting content. How do you feel after making this change?

3. **Support Network Map**: Draw a map of your support network. Include family, friends, mentors, and communities. Reflect on the strength of these connections and consider ways to strengthen them. Are there any gaps in your network that you could fill?

4. **Negative Influence Reflection**: Identify at least three negative influences in your life. Write down specific steps you can take to set boundaries and minimize their impact. How do you feel about implementing these changes?

5. **Space Makeover Plan**: Choose a space where you spend a lot of time and create a plan to declutter, organize, and personalize it. How can you make this space more conducive to your well-being and productivity?

By actively shaping your environment, both social and physical, you can create a supportive foundation that nurtures your growth and helps you reach your potential. Remember, a supportive environment is not built overnight—it requires ongoing effort and adjustment. But with each positive change, you'll find yourself closer to achieving the life you envision.

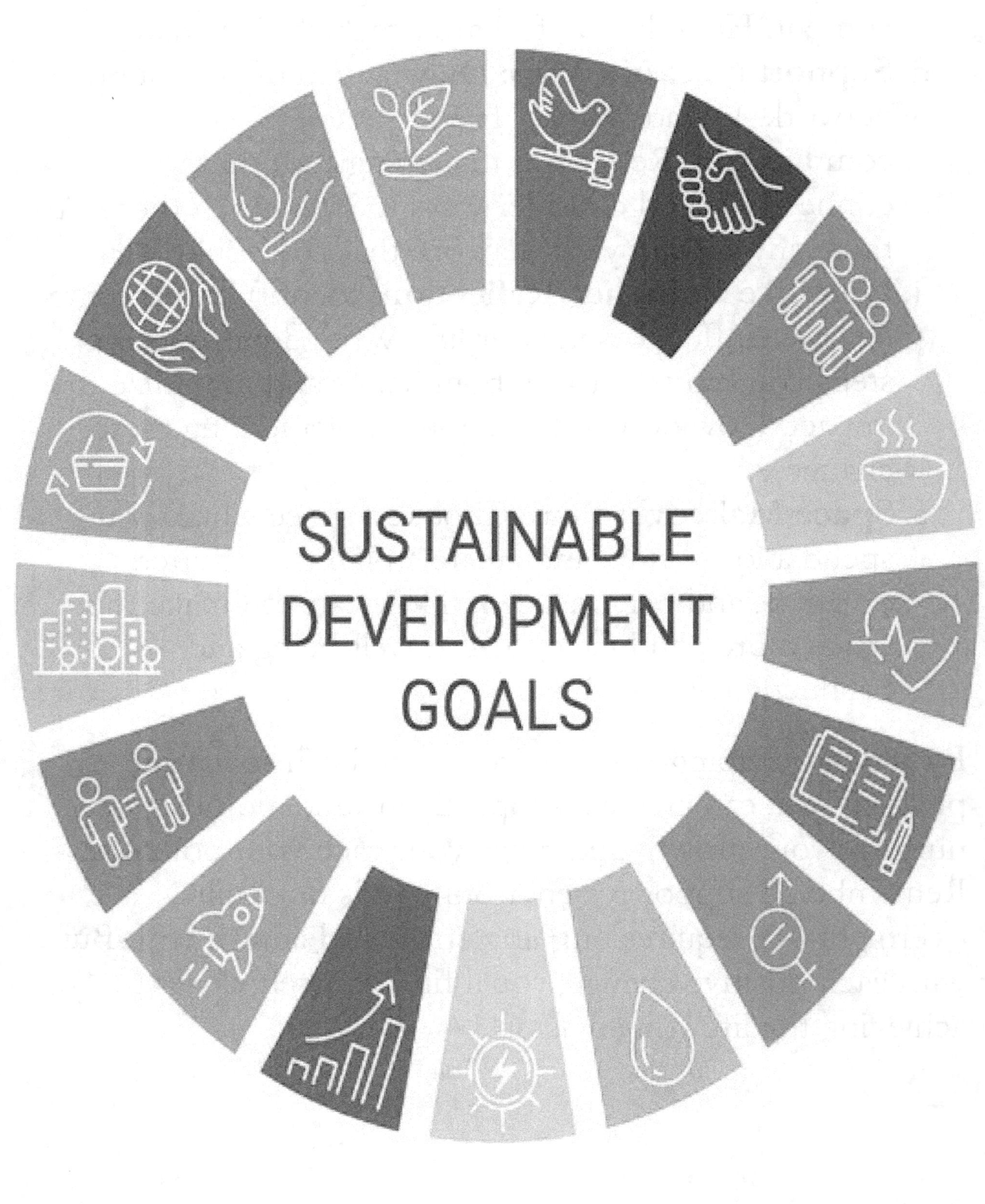

SUSTAINABLE
DEVELOPMENT
GOALS

Chapter 8: Sustaining Growth and Success

Introduction

Achieving personal growth and success is a significant milestone, but maintaining that growth and ensuring long-term success is where the real challenge lies. In this chapter, we will explore strategies for sustaining your progress, continuing to grow, and celebrating your successes in a way that fuels further achievements.

Sustaining growth requires continuous effort and adaptability. It's about building on the foundation you've already established, adjusting your strategies as needed, and maintaining the motivation that propelled you forward. By implementing the techniques discussed in this chapter, you'll be better equipped to ensure that your journey of growth and success remains dynamic and fulfilling.

The Importance of Sustaining Growth

Maintaining growth is crucial for several reasons:

1. **Long-Term Fulfillment**: True success is not a destination but a journey. Sustaining growth ensures that you continue to find fulfillment and purpose in your endeavors.
2. **Adapting to Change**: The world is constantly evolving, and so are your goals and challenges.

Sustained growth helps you adapt to these changes effectively.

3. **Continuous Improvement**: Growth is not a one-time achievement but an ongoing process. Sustaining it ensures that you are always moving towards becoming a better version of yourself.

Strategies for Sustaining Growth

1. Set New Goals

Once you achieve a goal, it's essential to set new ones to keep progressing. New goals provide direction and motivation. They should be:

- **Specific**: Clearly defined and measurable.
- **Challenging**: Push you out of your comfort zone.
- **Attainable**: Realistic yet ambitious.

  Example: If your goal was to complete a certification, your next goal might be to apply the new skills in a real-world project or pursue advanced training.

2. Continue Learning

Adopt a mindset of lifelong learning. Stay curious and open to acquiring new knowledge and skills. This can include:

- **Reading Books**: Stay updated with the latest in your field.

- **Attending Workshops**: Participate in seminars and workshops to enhance your skills.
- **Networking**: Engage with peers and mentors to exchange ideas and learn from their experiences.

Example: Enroll in online courses or attend industry conferences to stay ahead in your field.

3. Review and Reflect Regularly

Periodic self-reflection is key to understanding your progress and making necessary adjustments. Regular reviews help you:

- **Assess Progress**: Evaluate what's working and what's not.
- **Celebrate Successes**: Acknowledge and reward yourself for achievements.
- **Identify Areas for Improvement**: Determine where you need to focus your efforts.

Example: Set aside time each month to review your goals, progress, and any adjustments needed.

4. Maintain a Positive Mindset

A positive mindset is crucial for overcoming challenges and sustaining success. To maintain positivity:

- **Practice Gratitude**: Regularly acknowledge and appreciate the good things in your life.

- **Visualize Success**: Keep a clear vision of your goals and the benefits of achieving them.
- **Surround Yourself with Positivity**: Engage with supportive people who uplift and encourage you.

  Example: Start a gratitude journal where you record things you are thankful for each day.

5. Build a Support Network

A strong support network can provide encouragement, advice, and accountability. Cultivate relationships with:

- **Mentors**: Seek guidance from experienced individuals in your field.
- **Peers**: Connect with others who share similar goals and challenges.
- **Friends and Family**: Lean on loved ones for support and motivation.

  Example: Join professional organizations or groups related to your interests.

6. Embrace Flexibility

Flexibility allows you to adapt to changing circumstances and stay resilient. To embrace flexibility:

- **Be Open to Change**: Accept that your plans may need to adjust based on new information or circumstances.

- **Develop Problem-Solving Skills**: Enhance your ability to find solutions to unforeseen challenges.

  Example: When faced with unexpected changes, focus on how you can adapt rather than resisting the change.

7. Celebrate Milestones

Celebrating your achievements reinforces your motivation and commitment. Make sure to:

- **Recognize Small Wins**: Celebrate even minor successes to maintain enthusiasm.
- **Reflect on Achievements**: Take time to acknowledge the effort and progress you've made.

  Example: Treat yourself to something special or share your success with your support network.

Practical Exercise: Creating a Growth Plan

1. **Set a New Goal**: Identify a new goal that aligns with your current interests and aspirations. Make sure it is specific, challenging, and attainable.
2. **Develop a Learning Plan**: Create a plan for continuous learning. List resources, courses, or activities that will help you stay informed and skilled.
3. **Schedule Regular Reviews**: Set up a schedule for reviewing your progress. This could be monthly or quarterly, depending on your needs.

4. **Identify Support Sources**: Make a list of people who can support you in achieving your new goal. This might include mentors, peers, or family members.
5. **Create a Celebration Plan**: Plan how you will celebrate milestones and achievements. This could be as simple as a personal reward or a celebration with others.

Reflection Questions

1. What new goals can I set that align with my current aspirations?
2. What areas of knowledge or skills do I need to develop further to continue growing?
3. How often should I review my progress and what criteria will I use to assess it?
4. Who can support me in achieving my new goals, and how can I reach out to them?
5. How will I celebrate my milestones and achievements to stay motivated?

<u>Conclusion</u>

As we draw to the end of "Elevate Your Potential: A Guide to Personal Growth and Success," it's time to reflect on the journey we've embarked on together. From understanding the essence of your potential to implementing practical strategies for personal and professional growth, this book has been a roadmap to help you realize and harness the power within you.

Reflecting on Your Journey

Think back to the beginning of this book. You started by exploring the concept of potential—what it means and why it matters. You've learned about the importance of mindset, the art of goal-setting, and the science behind building lasting habits. You've confronted obstacles, leveraged your strengths, and created an environment that supports your growth.

Each chapter has been designed to offer you actionable advice and real-world examples, but the true success of this journey lies in your ability to put these insights into practice. It's not enough to merely understand these concepts; the real transformation happens when you actively apply them to your life.

The Path Forward

Personal growth is not a destination but a continuous journey. The principles and strategies discussed in this book are tools to guide you, but the path to success requires ongoing effort, reflection, and adaptation. Here are a few key takeaways to keep in mind as you move forward:

1. **Embrace Lifelong Learning**: Growth is a never-ending process. Stay curious, seek new knowledge, and be open to evolving. The more you learn, the more you grow.
2. **Adapt and Adjust**: Life is full of changes and challenges. Be flexible and willing to adjust your plans as needed. Adaptability is a crucial component of sustained success.
3. **Celebrate Your Achievements**: Recognize and celebrate your milestones, no matter how small. Each step forward is progress and deserves acknowledgment.
4. **Stay Resilient**: Setbacks are a natural part of the journey. Use them as learning opportunities and stay resilient in the face of adversity. Your ability to bounce back will determine your long-term success.

Continuing the Journey

As you continue on your path, remember that the journey of personal growth is uniquely yours. No one else can walk it for you, but you have the power to shape it. Use the tools and insights from this book as a foundation, and build upon them with your own experiences and discoveries.

Create a personal growth plan that reflects your goals, values, and aspirations. Regularly review and adjust it to stay aligned with your evolving vision. Surround yourself with supportive people who inspire and challenge you, and seek out resources that further your development.

Final Thoughts

You have within you the potential to achieve greatness and live a fulfilling life. By applying the principles from this book, you're taking an important step toward unlocking that potential. Believe in yourself, stay committed to your goals, and embrace the journey with an open heart and mind.

The world is full of opportunities waiting for you to seize them. Your potential is not limited by external circumstances but by your own willingness to strive for more. As you move forward, remember that you are capable of incredible things, and the best is yet to come.

Thank you for joining me on this journey. I hope this book has inspired you to take action, explore your potential, and pursue a path of personal growth and success. Here's to your continued growth, fulfillment, and the incredible journey ahead.

<u>Resources and Further Reading</u>

As you embark on your journey of personal growth and success, having access to valuable resources can provide additional insights, strategies, and motivation. Below, you'll find a curated list of books, articles, and tools that can complement the concepts discussed in "Elevate Your Potential: A Guide to Personal Growth and Success."

Books for Personal Growth and Success

1. **"Retail Revolution: The Ultimate Guide to Starting Your Wholesale and Retail Business" by Arya Gupta**
   - For those interested in the retail and wholesale business sector, this comprehensive guide offers practical advice on starting and growing a business. It covers everything from market analysis to operational strategies, providing valuable insights for aspiring entrepreneurs.

2. **"Atomic Habits: An Easy & Proven Way to Build Good Habits & Break Bad Ones" by James Clear**
   - This book provides a comprehensive guide on how to develop habits that stick and break those that don't. James Clear offers practical strategies for making small changes that lead to significant improvements over time.

3. **"Mindset: The New Psychology of Success" by Carol S. Dweck**
   - Carol Dweck explores the concept of mindset and its impact on our success. This book distinguishes between a fixed mindset and a growth mindset, offering insights on how to cultivate the latter to achieve personal and professional goals.
4. **"Grit: The Power of Passion and Perseverance" by Angela Duckworth**
   - Angela Duckworth examines the role of grit in achieving long-term goals. Her research highlights how passion and perseverance are key factors in success, providing actionable advice on how to develop these qualities.
5. **"The 7 Habits of Highly Effective People: Powerful Lessons in Personal Change" by Stephen R. Covey**
   - Stephen Covey's classic work outlines seven habits that can transform personal and professional effectiveness. This book offers practical advice on time management, goal setting, and interpersonal relationships.
6. **"Daring Greatly: How the Courage to Be Vulnerable Transforms the Way We Live, Love, Parent, and Lead" by Brené Brown**
   - Brené Brown delves into the concept of vulnerability and its role in building meaningful connections and achieving personal growth. Her

insights encourage readers to embrace vulnerability as a source of strength.

7. **"The Power of Now: A Guide to Spiritual Enlightenment" by Eckhart Tolle**
   - Eckhart Tolle's book focuses on the importance of living in the present moment. It provides a spiritual perspective on achieving inner peace and personal growth through mindfulness.
8. **"Start with Why: How Great Leaders Inspire Everyone to Take Action" by Simon Sinek**
   - Simon Sinek explores the concept of "why" and its role in inspiring action and leadership. This book is particularly useful for understanding how purpose-driven goals can lead to greater success and fulfillment.

Articles and Online Resources

1. **"The Science of Setting Goals" - Psychology Today**
   - An article that explores the psychology behind goal setting and offers practical tips for creating and achieving goals.
2. **"The Benefits of Mindfulness Meditation" - Harvard Health Publishing**
   - This article discusses the various benefits of mindfulness meditation, including its impact on mental health and overall well-being.
3. **"How to Develop a Growth Mindset" - MindTools**

- An online resource that provides actionable strategies for developing a growth mindset and overcoming challenges.

4. **"Effective Strategies for Overcoming Procrastination" - Forbes**
   - An article offering practical advice on how to tackle procrastination and improve productivity.

Tools and Apps

1. **Habitica**
   - An app that gamifies habit tracking and goal setting. It turns your daily tasks and habits into a role-playing game, making personal development more engaging and motivating.
2. **Headspace**
   - A popular app for mindfulness and meditation. It offers guided meditation sessions to help reduce stress and improve mental clarity.
3. **Trello**
   - A project management tool that helps you organize tasks and projects using boards and lists. It's useful for planning and tracking progress toward your goals.
4. **Evernote**
   - An app for note-taking and organization. It helps you keep track of ideas, plans, and to-do lists, making it easier to stay organized and focused.
   -

5. **Coursera and edX**
    - Online platforms offering courses on a variety of
      subjects, including personal development,
      leadership, and productivity. They provide access
      to high-quality content from reputable institutions.

Final Thoughts

These resources are meant to complement the insights and
strategies shared in "Elevate Your Potential: A Guide to
Personal Growth and Success." Whether you're looking to
build new habits, overcome challenges, or achieve specific
goals, these books, articles, and tools can provide valuable
support and inspiration.

Remember, personal growth is a continuous journey, and
the quest for success is uniquely personal. Explore these
resources, stay curious, and keep striving to unlock your full
potential. Your path to personal development is uniquely
your own, and every step you take brings you closer to
achieving your dreams.

About the Author

Arya Gupta is a passionate advocate for personal growth and self-improvement. With a background in Artificial Intelligence and Data Science, Arya combines analytical thinking with a deep understanding of human potential. Currently pursuing a B.Tech at Arya College of Engineering and IT, Arya brings a unique perspective to the realm of personal development, blending technical knowledge with practical strategies for success.

Arya's journey into the world of personal development was inspired by a desire to overcome personal challenges and unlock untapped potential. This journey led to the creation of "Elevate Your Potential: A Guide to Personal Growth and Success," a comprehensive guide designed to help others achieve their dreams and live fulfilling lives.

In addition to their work in personal development, Arya is also an entrepreneur. They founded an online wholesale and retail business, Manabhavan Industries, demonstrating a commitment to business growth and innovation. Arya's first book, "Retail Revolution: The Ultimate Guide to Starting Your Wholesale and Retail Business," provides valuable insights for aspiring entrepreneurs looking to break into the retail industry.

Arya believes in the power of continuous learning and self-improvement. They are dedicated to helping others discover their strengths, set meaningful goals, and navigate the path to success. Through writing, speaking, and mentoring, Arya aims to inspire and empower individuals to reach their full potential.

When not writing or working on business ventures, Arya enjoys exploring new technologies, reading, and spending time with family and friends and she is always looking for new ways to contribute to their community.

\

Call to Action

Thank you for taking the time to read "Elevate Your Potential: A Guide to Personal Growth and Success." I hope this book has provided you with valuable insights and practical strategies to enhance your personal and professional life.

If you enjoyed this book and found it helpful, here are a few ways you can continue your journey and stay connected:

1. **Read My Other Book**: Check out "Retail Revolution: The Ultimate Guide to Starting Your Wholesale and Retail Business" for practical advice on starting and growing a successful retail business. It's filled with actionable tips and real-world examples that can help you turn your entrepreneurial dreams into reality.
2. **Visit My Website**: For more resources, articles, and updates on my latest projects egarding business, visit Manabhavan Industries. Here, you'll find additional content to support your journey towards growth and business success.
3. **Connect on Social Media**: Follow me on social media to stay updated on new releases, upcoming events, and daily inspiration:
   - **LinkedIn**: https://www.linkedin.com/in/arya-gupta-71b00631b/
   - **Instagram**: @i_aryaguptaa
4. **Share Your Success Story**: I'd love to hear how this book has impacted your life. Share your success stories, feedback, or questions by reaching out via my social media. Your experiences can inspire and motivate others on their journey.
5. **Leave a Review**: If you found this book valuable, please consider leaving a review on Amazon or your favorite book retailer's website. Your feedback helps me improve and reach more readers who can benefit from these insights.